FATTY LIVER DIET COOKBOOK FOR BEGINNERS

Ultimate Guide To Nourish Your Liver And Rejuvenate Your Body With Delicious And Nutrient-packed Recipes | 7-Days Meal Plan Included

Corey Pearce

Copyright © 2023 Corey Pearce

OTHER BOOKS BY THIS AUTHOR

Table of Contents

Chapter 1:
Introduction

In the hectic pace of modern life, health frequently takes a second place to the confusion of everyday responsibilities. Yet, tucked within our bodies, the liver works relentlessly, a quiet hero in the symphony of our health. As a dietitian, I've seen firsthand the transformational effect of diet on general health, and one organ that demands our attention is the liver.

Consider the following: A crucial organ that discreetly navigates our body's intricacies, filtering out poisons, metabolizing nutrients, and coordinating processes that keep us alive. Consider it burdened, suffering under the weight of an increasingly common modern ailment - fatty liver disease. This is the hidden catastrophe that affects millions, frequently going unnoticed by its victims until symptoms appear.

This understanding motivated my determination to explore the complexities of liver health and provide a ray of hope via the pages of this Fatty Liver Diet Cookbook for Beginners. I've walked with people dealing with the effects of fatty liver disease, experiencing their journeys from uncertainty to clarity, from despair to empowerment.

This book is more than simply a compilation of recipes; it's a lifeline for individuals looking for a method to restore their liver health. I welcome you to read the stories of those who have successfully navigated the maze of fatty liver issues and emerged stronger and healthier on the other side. Their tales speak to the possibilities of transformation through deliberate, tasty, and healthy choices.

Within these pages, you'll find a culinary voyage - a trip that combines the beauty of food with the science of healing. The dishes presented here are more than just ingredients; they are instruments for resilience, with each mouthful a step toward renewing the unsung hero inside.

As you begin on this culinary adventure, remember that this is more than just a cookbook; it is your guide to a flourishing life. A life in which your liver thrives, your body thrives, and every meal is a celebration of well-being. Join me on this gourmet trip where food meets change and the path to a healthier you begins with each tasty chapter.

So, dear reader, let this book be your guide, ally, and inspiration. Allow its pages to tell a story of health, healing, and the tremendous influence of decisions. Your liver deserves the finest, and through the artistry of a well-crafted diet, you wield the brush that paints the canvas of your vivid future. Welcome to the Fatty Liver Diet Cookbook for Beginners, where the tale of your health begins afresh.

Exploring the Importance of Dietary Options:

In this exposé, we address the secret issue that affects millions of people: fatty liver disease. This illness, which is frequently undiscovered until symptoms appear, emphasizes the vital role that our diets play in supporting liver function. It's not just about the food we eat; it's a story about empowerment, where each mouthful becomes a chance to reinforce and refresh.

We dig into the subtle dance between diet and liver function as we peel back the layers of understanding. What foods we eat feed or stress this crucial organ? What can we learn from individuals who have successfully navigated the maze of liver health? Dietary choices become a compass, directing us along a route where educated judgments pave the way for long-term well-being.

How to Get a Healthier Liver:

This book is more than just a collection of recipes; it's a roadmap to a healthy liver. We start on a journey where culinary choices become a transformational force via immersive storytelling, real-life anecdotes, and expert insights. Whether you are dealing with the difficulties of fatty liver disease or looking for preventative measures, this book provides a route - a path that navigates past fear and confusion, bringing you to a regenerated liver and a more vibrant existence.

Allow the significance of your food choices to reverberate as we embark on this journey. Your route to a healthier liver is not a strict routine, but rather a celebration of nutritious, tasty, and deliberate choices. It's time to see the possibilities in every meal, understanding that every mouthful contributes to the story of your health. Welcome to a journey in which your nutritional choices act as a catalyst for a more vibrant, resilient, and refreshed self.

THIS PAGE WAS INTENTIONALLY LEFT BLANK

Chapter 2: Understanding the Fundamentals of the Fatty Liver Diet

The Nutritional Role in Fatty Liver Management

Your path to a healthy liver begins with a thorough awareness of the critical role diet plays in fatty liver management. Investigate the delicate dance between what you eat and how it affects your liver function. Examine the following crucial points:

1. Macronutrient Balance:
- Discover the significance of a well-balanced diet that includes carbs, proteins, and fats.
- Investigate how the proper balance can improve liver function and assist in the prevention and treatment of fatty liver disease.

2. The Influence of Sugar and Carbohydrates:
- Discover the negative consequences of too much sugar and processed carbs on liver function.
- Learn about the link between high-fructose corn syrup and the development of fatty liver disease.

3. The Power of Healthy Fats:
- Learn about the importance of vital fatty acids like omega-3 and omega-6 in liver function.
- Investigate sources of healthy fats and how to include them into your diet for optimal liver function.

4. Protein Contribution: Recognize the importance of protein in the fatty liver diet.
- Discover the significance of protein in liver cell regeneration and overall liver wellbeing.

Determining Trigger Foods and Suspects

Navigate the nutritional terrain by recognizing items that can either nourish or hurt your liver. Investigate the following critical elements:

1. Hidden Culprits:
- Uncover the seemingly harmless items that may lead to fatty liver disease.
- Be mindful of hidden sugars, processed meals, and high-fat selections that might harm your liver.

2. The Impact of Alcohol:
- Identify the link between alcohol intake and fatty liver disease.
- Discover acceptable alcohol limits and the need of abstinence for persons suffering from fatty liver disease.

3. Processed and Fried Foods:
- Determine the contribution of processed and fried foods to liver fat buildup.
- Investigate better cooking methods and alternatives to shield your liver from potentially dangerous food choices.

4. Salt and Sodium Awareness:
- Understand the link between excessive salt consumption and liver issues.
- Investigate methods for lowering salt in your diet while still eating tasty and enjoyable meals.

THIS PAGE WAS INTENTIONALLY LEFT BLANK

Chapter 3: How to Begin Your Fatty Liver Diet

Evaluate Your Current Diet

Beginning your road to a liver-friendly diet requires a thorough review of your existing eating patterns. To examine and understand your food trends, take the following steps:

1. Food Diary:
- Start by keeping a comprehensive food diary in which you note everything you eat and drink.
- Take careful note of your portion amounts, meal times, and any snacks you take throughout the day.

2. Nutrient Analysis:
- Examine the nutritional content of your meals, paying close attention to calorie, fat, sugar, and salt consumption.
- Determine if your diet is deficient in critical nutrients or excessive in other areas.

3. Consulting a practitioner:
- Consult a healthcare practitioner or a certified dietician for advice.
- Discuss your eating habits, health objectives, and any specific fatty liver disease concerns with your doctor.

4. Understanding Triggers:
- Identify particular items or dietary patterns that may be related to liver stress.
- Recognize triggers like too much sugar, processed foods, or high-fat meals that may need to be modified.

Transition Gradually to Liver-Friendly Eating

Making long-term food adjustments requires a gradual and sustained shift. To ease into a liver-friendly eating regimen, use the following strategies:

1. Set Realistic Goals:
- Based on your dietary evaluation, set attainable short-term and long-term goals.
- Break down larger ambitions into digestible steps to ensure a more sustainable transition.

2. Slow Reduction of Culprits:
- Rather than making radical adjustments all at once, gradually lower your intake of recognized trigger foods.
- This method reduces the probability of feeling overwhelmed while also increasing adherence to the new eating plan.

3. Incorporate Whole Foods:
- Include nutrient-dense whole foods including fruits, vegetables, lean meats, and whole grains in your diet.
- Play with different flavors and textures to make the transition more delightful and fulfilling.

4. Meal Preparation and Planning:
- Plan your meals ahead of time to guarantee a well-balanced and liver-friendly diet.
- Participate in meal preparation, experimenting with new dishes that correspond to your dietary objectives.

5. Hydration Awareness:
- Incorporate water into your daily routine to emphasize the necessity of being hydrated.
- Limit your intake of sugary drinks and alcohol in favor of healthier choices.

THIS PAGE WAS INTENTIONALLY LEFT BLANK

Chapter 4: Fatty Liver Diet Shopping Tips

Navigating Grocery Stores with a Purpose

Efficient and deliberate food shopping is essential to keeping a healthy fatty liver diet. To explore grocery shops with purpose, use the following advice:

1. Plan Before You Go:
- Make a shopping list based on your weekly meal plans.
- A concise list allows you to stay focused and prevent impulse purchases.

2. Shop the Perimeter:
- Look for fresh vegetables, lean proteins, and dairy on the grocery store's outside aisles.
- Spend as little time as possible in the processed food aisles to limit your exposure to harmful contaminants.

3. Select Colorful Produce:
- Prioritize a range of colorful fruits and vegetables to guarantee a broad spectrum of nutrients.

- Choose fresh, frozen, or canned foods free of added sugars and hazardous preservatives.

4. Select Lean Proteins:
- Place poultry, fish, tofu, and beans in your shopping cart.
- Limit processed and fatty meats, which may add to liver stress.

Checking Labels for Liver-Boosting Ingredients

Understanding food labels is an important skill to have if you want to follow a liver-boosting diet. Consider the following advice:

1. Check for Added Sugars:
- Examine the ingredient list for hidden sugars disguised as sucrose, high fructose corn syrup, or agave nectar.
- Choose goods with minimal to no added sugars, especially those branded "low-fat" or "diet."

2. Mindful Fat Choices:
- Select foods high in healthy fats, such as avocados, almonds, and olive oil.

- Limit saturated and trans fats, which are typically present in processed foods and some cooking oils.

3. Sodium Awareness:
- Check the sodium level of packaged goods, since too much salt might contribute to liver problems.
- Choose low-sodium or sodium-free options, then season with herbs and spices.

4. Whole Grain Selection:
- Look for whole grains in bread, pasta, and rice selections.
- Choose items with "whole" or "whole grain" as the first ingredient for more fiber and minerals.

5. Avoid Artificial additions:
- Avoid foods that include artificial additions, colorings, or preservatives.
- Select less processed products to limit the consumption of chemicals that may stress the liver.

THIS PAGE WAS INTENTIONALLY LEFT BLANK

Chapter 5: Easy Meal Planning

Creating Balanced Menus for Healthy Fatty Liver

Creating well-balanced dinners is a critical component of following a fatty liver-friendly diet. Follow these suggestions to guarantee that your meals are not only delicious but also beneficial to your liver:

1. Broad Nutrient Intake:
- Incorporate a range of fruits, vegetables, whole grains, lean meats, and healthy fats into your meals to achieve a broad array of nutrients.
- To keep your meals interesting and pleasant, experiment with varied colors, textures, and flavors.

2. Prioritize Lean Proteins:
- Include lean protein sources in your meals such as fish, chicken, tofu, and lentils.
- To reduce additional fats, choose cooking methods such as grilling, baking, or steaming.

3. Embrace Whole Grains:
- Choose whole grains over refined grains such as quinoa, brown rice, and whole wheat bread.
- Whole grains include fiber and minerals that are good to liver function.

4. Healthy Fats in Moderation:
- Include healthy fat sources such as avocados, almonds, and olive oil in reasonable quantities.
- Maintain a healthy fat intake without overburdening the liver.

5. Portion Variety:
- Observe portion proportions to avoid overeating and to aid in weight control.
- Use smaller plates and bowls to provide the idea of a bigger meal while keeping quantities under control.

Portion Control and Timing Techniques

Strategic portion management and thoughtful meal scheduling are important components of a healthy fatty liver diet. Consider the following approaches:

1. Regular, Balanced Meals:
- Attempt to have three balanced meals each day, plus snacks as required.
- Consistent eating patterns aid in blood sugar regulation and general metabolic health.

2. Listen to Hunger signs:
- Become aware of your body's hunger and fullness signs.
- Instead of eating for boredom or emotional reasons, focus on fueling your body when it is truly hungry.

3. Controlled Serving Sizes:
- Control serving sizes using measurement equipment or visual signals.
- Avoid consuming huge quantities, particularly in restaurants where servings may be bigger than necessary.

4. Smart Snacking:
- Choose nutrient-dense snacks in between meals to keep your energy levels up.
- Choose fruits, veggies, yogurt, or a handful of nuts.

5. Mindful Eating Practices:
- Savor each mouthful and pay attention to the flavors and sensations of your meal to practice mindful eating.
- To enhance awareness during meals, avoid distractions such as TV or technological gadgets.

7 Days Meal Planning for fatty liver diet

DAY 1:
Breakfast: Scrambled Eggs with Spinach and Tomatoes

INGREDIENTS:
- 2 eggs
- Handful of fresh spinach
- Cherry tomatoes, halved
- Salt and pepper to taste
- Olive oil for cooking

INSTRUCTIONS:
1. Heat olive oil in a pan over medium heat.
2. Add cherry tomatoes and spinach to the pan, sauté until spinach wilts.
3. Whisk eggs in a bowl and pour over the vegetables.
4. Scramble the eggs until fully cooked.

5. Season with salt and pepper to taste.

Grilled Chicken Salad:

INGREDIENTS:
- Grilled chicken breast, sliced
- Mixed salad greens (lettuce, arugula, spinach)
- Cherry tomatoes, halved
- Red onion, thinly sliced
- Vinaigrette dressing (olive oil, balsamic vinegar, Dijon mustard, honey)
- Salt and pepper to taste

INSTRUCTIONS:
1. In a large bowl, combine mixed greens, cherry tomatoes, and red onion.
2. Top the salad with grilled chicken slices.
3. In a small bowl, whisk together olive oil, balsamic vinegar, Dijon mustard, and honey for the vinaigrette.
4. Drizzle the vinaigrette over the salad and toss gently.
5. Season with salt and pepper to taste.

Quinoa on the Side:
- Cook quinoa according to package instructions.

Snack: Greek Yogurt with a Handful of Berries
INGREDIENTS:
- Greek yogurt
- Mixed berries (blueberries, strawberries, raspberries)

INSTRUCTIONS:
1. Spoon Greek yogurt into a bowl.
2. Top with a handful of mixed berries.

Dinner: Steamed Broccoli and Cauliflower
INGREDIENTS:
- Broccoli florets
- Cauliflower florets
- Lemon juice
- Olive oil
- Salt and pepper to taste

INSTRUCTIONS:
1. Steam broccoli and cauliflower until tender-crisp.
2. In a bowl, toss the steamed vegetables with lemon juice and olive oil.

3. Season with salt and pepper to taste.

DAY 2:

Breakfast: Oatmeal topped with Sliced Bananas and a Sprinkle of Chia Seeds, Almond Milk

Oatmeal topped with Sliced Bananas and a Sprinkle of Chia Seeds:
INGREDIENTS:
- 1/2 cup rolled oats
- 1 cup almond milk
- Sliced bananas
- Chia seeds

INSTRUCTIONS:
1. Cook oats with almond milk according to package instructions.
2. Top the oatmeal with sliced bananas.
3. Sprinkle chia seeds over the top.

Almond Milk:
- Pour a glass of almond milk to accompany your oatmeal.

Lunch: Turkey and Avocado Wrap with Whole Grain Tortilla, Mixed Green Salad

Turkey and Avocado Wrap with Whole Grain Tortilla:
INGREDIENTS:
- Whole grain tortilla
- Sliced turkey breast
- Avocado, sliced
- Lettuce leaves

INSTRUCTIONS:
1. Lay the whole grain tortilla flat.
2. Layer with sliced turkey, avocado, and lettuce leaves.
3. Roll the tortilla into a wrap.

Mixed Green Salad:
- Prepare a side salad with a mix of greens such as lettuce, spinach, and arugula.
- Add cherry tomatoes and a light vinaigrette dressing.

Snack: Carrot and Cucumber Sticks with Hummus
INGREDIENTS:
- Carrot sticks
- Cucumber sticks

- Hummus

INSTRUCTIONS:
1. Cut carrots and cucumbers into sticks.
2. Dip the sticks into hummus before enjoying.

Dinner: Stir-fried Tofu with Colorful Vegetables (Bell Peppers, Broccoli, Carrots)

INGREDIENTS:
- Firm tofu, cubed
- Bell peppers (assorted colors), sliced
- Broccoli florets
- Carrots, julienned
- Soy sauce
- Sesame oil
- Garlic, minced
- Ginger, grated
- Green onions, chopped (for garnish)
- Cooked brown rice (optional, for serving)

INSTRUCTIONS:
1. In a wok or skillet, heat sesame oil over medium heat.
2. Add minced garlic and grated ginger, sauté until fragrant.
3. Add cubed tofu and stir-fry until golden brown.

4. Add sliced bell peppers, broccoli florets, and julienned carrots. Continue to stir-fry until vegetables are tender-crisp.
5. Drizzle soy sauce over the tofu and vegetables, toss to combine.
6. Serve over cooked brown rice if desired and garnish with chopped green onions.

DAY 3:

Breakfast: Smoothie with Spinach, Banana, Berries, and Almond Milk

INGREDIENTS:
- Handful of fresh spinach
- 1 banana
- Mixed berries (blueberries, strawberries, raspberries)
- 1 cup almond milk

INSTRUCTIONS:
1. In a blender, combine fresh spinach, banana, mixed berries, and almond milk.
2. Blend until smooth and creamy.

Lunch: Lentil Soup

INGREDIENTS:
- 1 cup dry lentils, rinsed
- Vegetable broth
- Carrots, diced
- Celery, diced

- Onion, chopped
- Garlic, minced
- Cumin, ground
- Coriander, ground
- Salt and pepper to taste

INSTRUCTIONS:
1. In a large pot, sauté onions and garlic until softened.
2. Add diced carrots and celery, cook until vegetables are tender.
3. Stir in lentils, cumin, coriander, salt, and pepper.
4. Pour in vegetable broth and bring to a simmer.
5. Cook until lentils are tender and flavors are well combined.

Snack: Handful of Mixed Nuts
INGREDIENTS:
- Mixed nuts (almonds, walnuts, pistachios, etc.)

INSTRUCTIONS:
- Grab a handful of mixed nuts for a satisfying and nutritious snack.

Dinner: Grilled Shrimp Skewers with Zucchini and Cherry Tomatoes

INGREDIENTS:
- Shrimp, peeled and deveined
- Zucchini, sliced
- Cherry tomatoes
- Olive oil
- Lemon juice
- Garlic, minced
- Paprika
- Salt and pepper to taste

INSTRUCTIONS:
1. In a bowl, combine shrimp, zucchini slices, cherry tomatoes, olive oil, lemon juice, minced garlic, paprika, salt, and pepper.
2. Thread shrimp, zucchini, and tomatoes onto skewers.
3. Grill skewers until shrimp are cooked and vegetables are tender.

DAY 4:

Breakfast: Greek Yogurt Parfait with Granola and Mixed Berries

INGREDIENTS:
- Greek yogurt
- Granola
- Mixed berries (blueberries, strawberries, raspberries)

- Honey (optional)

INSTRUCTIONS:
1. In a glass or bowl, layer Greek yogurt at the bottom.
2. Add a layer of granola on top of the yogurt.
3. Add a layer of mixed berries.
4. Repeat the layers until the glass or bowl is filled.
5. Drizzle honey on top if desired.

Lunch: Quinoa Salad with Chickpeas, Cherry Tomatoes, Cucumber, and Feta Cheese

INGREDIENTS:
- Cooked quinoa
- Chickpeas, drained and rinsed
- Cherry tomatoes, halved
- Cucumber, diced
- Feta cheese, crumbled
- Olive oil
- Balsamic vinegar
- Fresh basil, chopped
- Salt and pepper to taste

INSTRUCTIONS:
1. In a large bowl, combine cooked quinoa, chickpeas, cherry tomatoes, cucumber, and feta cheese.

2. Drizzle with olive oil and balsamic vinegar.
3. Add fresh basil, salt, and pepper to taste.
4. Toss the salad gently until well combined.

Snack: Sliced Pear with a Tablespoon of Almond Butter

INGREDIENTS:
- Pear, sliced
- Almond butter

INSTRUCTIONS:
- Slice a pear and serve it with a tablespoon of almond butter.

Dinner: Baked Chicken Breast with Rosemary and Garlic

INGREDIENTS:
- Chicken breast
- Fresh rosemary, chopped
- Garlic, minced
- Olive oil
- Lemon juice
- Salt and pepper to taste

INSTRUCTIONS:
1. Preheat the oven to 375°F (190°C).
2. Place chicken breasts in a baking dish.
3. In a bowl, mix chopped rosemary, minced garlic, olive oil, lemon juice, salt, and pepper.

4. Rub the mixture over the chicken breasts.

5. Bake in the preheated oven until the chicken is cooked through.

DAY 5:

Breakfast: Whole Grain Pancakes with Fresh Berries and a Drizzle of Honey

INGREDIENTS:
- Whole grain pancake mix
- Fresh berries (blueberries, strawberries, raspberries)
- Honey

INSTRUCTIONS:

1. Prepare whole grain pancakes according to the package instructions.

2. Top the pancakes with fresh berries.

3. Drizzle honey over the pancakes.

Lunch: Spinach and Feta-Stuffed Chicken Breast

INGREDIENTS:
- Chicken breast
- Fresh spinach leaves
- Feta cheese, crumbled
- Olive oil
- Garlic, minced
- Salt and pepper to taste

INSTRUCTIONS:
1. Preheat the oven to 375°F (190°C).
2. Butterfly the chicken breast.
3. In a bowl, mix fresh spinach, crumbled feta, minced garlic, salt, and pepper.
4. Stuff the chicken breast with the spinach and feta mixture.
5. Secure with toothpicks if needed.
6. Bake in the preheated oven until the chicken is cooked through.

Snack: Cottage Cheese with Pineapple Chunks

INGREDIENTS:
- Cottage cheese
- Pineapple chunks

INSTRUCTIONS:
- Combine cottage cheese with pineapple chunks for a tasty and satisfying snack.

Dinner: Grilled Trout with Lemon and Dill

INGREDIENTS:
- Trout fillets
- Lemon, sliced
- Fresh dill, chopped
- Olive oil
- Salt and pepper to taste

INSTRUCTIONS:
1. Preheat the grill or grill pan.
2. Rub trout fillets with olive oil and season with salt, pepper, and chopped dill.
3. Place lemon slices on top of the fillets.
4. Grill until the fish is cooked through.

DAY 6:
Breakfast: Scrambled Tofu with Sautéed Mushrooms and Spinach
INGREDIENTS:
- Firm tofu, crumbled
- Mushrooms, sliced
- Fresh spinach leaves
- Olive oil
- Turmeric powder (for color)
- Salt and pepper to taste

INSTRUCTIONS:
1. In a pan, sauté sliced mushrooms in olive oil until tender.
2. Add crumbled tofu to the pan, sprinkle with turmeric powder for color.
3. Stir in fresh spinach leaves and cook until wilted.
4. Season with salt and pepper to taste.

Lunch: Turkey and Vegetable Stir-Fry with Brown Rice

INGREDIENTS:
- Lean turkey breast, sliced
- Mixed vegetables (bell peppers, broccoli, carrots), sliced
- Soy sauce
- Ginger, minced
- Garlic, minced
- Olive oil
- Cooked brown rice

INSTRUCTIONS:
1. Heat olive oil in a wok or skillet.
2. Stir-fry sliced turkey until cooked through.
3. Add minced ginger and garlic to the pan.
4. Add mixed vegetables and continue to stir-fry until vegetables are tender-crisp.
5. Pour soy sauce over the stir-fry and toss to combine.
6. Serve over cooked brown rice.

Snack: Sliced Mango with a Sprinkle of Chili Powder

INGREDIENTS:
- Ripe mango, sliced
- Chili powder

INSTRUCTIONS:
- Slice a ripe mango and sprinkle chili powder for a sweet and slightly spicy snack.

Dinner: Steamed Broccoli and Carrots
INGREDIENTS:
- Broccoli florets
- Carrots, sliced
- Lemon juice
- Olive oil
- Salt and pepper to taste

INSTRUCTIONS:
1. Steam broccoli florets and sliced carrots until tender-crisp.
2. In a bowl, toss steamed vegetables with lemon juice and olive oil.
3. Season with salt and pepper to taste.

DAY 7:

Breakfast: Chia Seed Pudding with Coconut Milk and Sliced Kiwi
INGREDIENTS:
- Chia seeds
- Coconut milk
- Maple syrup (optional, for sweetness)
- Vanilla extract (optional)
- Sliced kiwi (for topping)

INSTRUCTIONS:
1. In a bowl, mix chia seeds with coconut milk.
2. Add maple syrup and vanilla extract if desired, adjusting sweetness to taste.
3. Stir well and let it sit in the refrigerator for a few hours or overnight until it thickens.
4. Top with sliced kiwi before serving.

Lunch: Mixed Green Salad with Balsamic Vinaigrette

INGREDIENTS:
- Mixed salad greens (lettuce, arugula, spinach)
- Cherry tomatoes, halved
- Cucumber, sliced
- Red onion, thinly sliced
- Balsamic vinaigrette dressing
- Salt and pepper to taste

INSTRUCTIONS:
1. In a large bowl, combine mixed salad greens, cherry tomatoes, cucumber, and red onion.
2. Drizzle with balsamic vinaigrette dressing.
3. Toss the salad gently until well combined.
4. Season with salt and pepper to taste.

Snack: Celery Sticks with Hummus

INGREDIENTS:
- Celery sticks

- Hummus

INSTRUCTIONS:
- Dip celery sticks into hummus for a crunchy and satisfying snack.

Dinner: Baked Chicken Thighs with Lemon and Herbs

INGREDIENTS:
- Chicken thighs, bone-in and skin-on
- Lemon, sliced
- Fresh herbs (rosemary, thyme, oregano), chopped
- Garlic, minced
- Olive oil
- Salt and pepper to taste

INSTRUCTIONS:
1. Preheat the oven to 375°F (190°C).
2. In a bowl, mix chopped herbs, minced garlic, olive oil, salt, and pepper.
3. Rub the herb mixture over the chicken thighs.
4. Place lemon slices on top of the chicken.
5. Bake in the preheated oven until the chicken is cooked through and skin is crispy.

THIS PAGE WAS INTENTIONALLY LEFT BLANK

Chapter 6: Dive into Deliciousness: Fatty Liver-Friendly Recipes

Breakfast Bliss: Energizing Your Mornings

1. Oatmeal with Berries and Almond Milk

INGREDIENTS:
- 1/2 cup rolled oats
- 1 cup almond milk
- Mixed fruit (blueberries, strawberries, raspberries)

PREPARATION:
1. Cook rolled oats with almond milk until creamy.
2. Top with assorted berries.

NUTRITIONAL VALUE:
- High in fiber, antioxidants, and omega-3 fatty acids.

Cooking Time: 5-7 minutes.

2. Chia Seed Pudding Parfait

INGREDIENTS:
- 2 tbsp chia seeds
- 1 cup coconut milk
- Sliced kiwi
- Granola

PREPARATION:
1. Mix chia seeds with coconut milk and refrigerate until pudding-like consistency.
2. Layer chia seed pudding with sliced kiwi and granola.

NUTRITIONAL VALUE:
- Rich in fiber, healthful lipids, and vitamins.

Cooking Time: 2-4 hours (including refrigeration).

3. Greek Yogurt Bowl with Nuts and Honey

INGREDIENTS:
- 1 cup Greek yogurt
- Mixed nuts (almonds, walnuts)
- Honey

PREPARATION:
1. Spoon Greek yogurt into a dish.

2. Top with assorted almonds and a drizzle of honey.

NUTRITIONAL VALUE:
- High in protein, healthful lipids, and antioxidants.

Preparation Time: 5 minutes.

4. Spinach and Mushroom Egg Scramble
INGREDIENTS:
- 2 eggs
- Handful of raw spinach
- Sliced mushrooms

PREPARATION:
1. Whisk eggs and scramble with spinach and mushrooms.

NUTRITIONAL VALUE:
- High in protein, iron, and vitamins.

Cooking Time: 5 minutes.

5. Avocado and Tomato Whole Grain Toast
INGREDIENTS:
- 1 slice whole grain bread
- 1/2 avocado, pureed

- Sliced cherry tomatoes

PREPARATION:
1. Toast whole grain bread and distribute pureed avocado.
2. Top with diced cherry tomatoes.

NUTRITIONAL VALUE:
- Rich in fiber, healthful lipids, and micronutrients.

Cooking Time: 3-5 minutes.

6. Quinoa Breakfast Bowl
INGREDIENTS:
- 1/2 cup cooked quinoa
- Greek yogurt
- Fresh cherries
- Chopped nuts (almonds, pistachios)

PREPARATION:
1. Combine cooked quinoa with Greek yogurt.
2. Top with fresh berries and sliced almonds.

NUTRITIONAL VALUE:
- High in protein, fiber, and antioxidants.

Preparation Time: 10 minutes.

7. Cottage Cheese and Pineapple Parfait

INGREDIENTS:
- Cottage cheese
- Fresh pineapple pieces
- Granola

PREPARATION:
1. Layer cottage cheese with pineapple pieces and cereals.

NUTRITIONAL VALUE:
- Good source of protein, calcium, and vitamins.

Preparation Time: 5 minutes.

8. Sweet Potato and Turkey Sausage Hash

INGREDIENTS:
- Sweet potatoes, diced
- Turkey sausage, cut
- Spinach leaves

PREPARATION:
1. Sauté minced sweet potatoes and turkey sausage until heated.
2. Add spinach and simmer until wilted.

NUTRITIONAL VALUE:
- High in fiber, protein, and essential nutrients.

Cooking Time: 15 minutes.

9. Buckwheat Pancakes with Berry Compote
INGREDIENTS:
- 1/2 cup buckwheat flour
- 1/2 cup almond milk
- Mixed berries (for compote)

PREPARATION:
1. Mix buckwheat flour with almond milk to create batter.
2. Cook pancakes and garnish with a mixed berry compote.

NUTRITIONAL VALUE:
- Rich in fiber, antioxidants, and gluten-free.

Cooking Time: 10 minutes.

10. Fruit and Nut Smoothie Bowl
INGREDIENTS:
- Mixed frozen fruits (berries, banana)
- Almond milk
- Mixed nuts (almonds, walnuts)

PREPARATION:

1. Blend frozen fruits with almond milk until homogeneous.

2. Pour into a basin and garnish with assorted almonds.

NUTRITIONAL VALUE:

- High in vitamins, fiber, and healthful lipids.

Preparation Time: 5 minutes.

Lunchtime Delights: Nutrient-Packed Midday Meals

1. Grilled Salmon Salad

INGREDIENTS:

- 6 oz salmon fillet
- Mixed salad greens (2 cups)
- Cherry tomatoes, divided (1 cup)
- Cucumber, divided (1/2 cup)
- Olive oil (1 tbsp)
- Lemon juice (1 tbsp)
- Salt and pepper to flavor

PREPARATION:

1. Season salmon tenderloin with salt and pepper.

2. Grill salmon until cooked (about 4-5 minutes per side).
3. Toss salad greens, cherry tomatoes, and cucumber in a basin.
4. Top with seared salmon.
5. Drizzle with olive oil and lemon juice.

NUTRITIONAL VALUE:
- Protein: 30g - Healthy Fats: 10g
- Fiber: 5g

Cooking Time: 10 minutes

2. Quinoa and Vegetable Stir-Fry

INGREDIENTS:
- Cooked quinoa (1 cup)
- Broccoli florets (1 cup)
- Carrots, julienned (1/2 cup)
- Bell peppers, divided (1/2 cup)
- Tofu, diced (4 lb)
- Soy sauce (2 tbsp)
- Sesame oil (1 tbsp)
- Garlic, minced (1 tsp)

PREPARATION:
1. Heat sesame oil in a griddle.
2. Sauté garlic, add tofu, and stir-fry until golden.
3. Add broccoli, carrots, and bell peppers.

4. Stir in prepared quinoa.

5. Pour soy sauce and stir until well combined.

NUTRITIONAL VALUE:

- Protein: 15g
- Healthy Fats: 8g
- Fiber: 7g

Cooking Time: 15 minutes

3. Turkey and Spinach Wrap

INGREDIENTS:

- Whole grain tortilla (1)
- Lean minced turkey (4 oz)
- Fresh spinach leaves (1 cup)
- Avocado, diced (1/2)
- Greek yogurt (2 tbsp)
- Salsa (2 tbsp)

PREPARATION:

1. Cook minced turkey until browned.

2. Warm the whole grain tortilla.

3. Spread Greek yogurt on the tortilla.

4. Layer with cooked turkey, fresh spinach, avocado segments, and salsa.

5. Wrap and secure with toothpicks if required.

NUTRITIONAL VALUE:

- Protein: 20g - Healthy Fats: 10g

- Fiber: 6g

Cooking Time: 15 minutes

4. Vegetable and Lentil Soup

INGREDIENTS:
- Lentils, cleansed (1/2 cup)
- Carrots, minced (1/2 cup)
- Celery, diced (1/2 cup)
- Onion, minced (1/2 cup)
- Vegetable bouillon (2 pints)
- Garlic, minced (1 tsp)
- Bay fronds (2)
- Turmeric powder (1/2 tsp)

PREPARATION:
1. In a saucepan, sauté onions and garlic until translucent.
2. Add lentils, carrots, celery, and bay leaves.
3. Pour in vegetable broth and add turmeric powder.
4. Simmer until legumes are tender.

NUTRITIONAL VALUE:
- Protein: 12g
- Healthy Fats: 1g
- Fiber: 8g

Cooking Time: 30 minutes

5. Chicken and Quinoa Salad Bowl
INGREDIENTS:
- Grilled chicken breast, divided (6 lb)
- Cooked quinoa (1 cup)
- Mixed salad greens (2 gallons)
- Cherry tomatoes, divided (1 cup)
- Avocado, minced (1/2)
- Balsamic vinaigrette marinade (2 tbsp)

PREPARATION:
1. Arrange salad greens in a dish.
2. Top with sliced seared chicken, prepared quinoa, cherry tomatoes, and diced avocado.
3. Drizzle with balsamic vinaigrette marinade.

NUTRITIONAL VALUE:
- Protein: 30g - Healthy Fats: 15g
- Fiber: 7g

Cooking Time: 20 minutes

6. Sweet Potato and Chickpea Salad
INGREDIENTS:
- Roasted sweet potatoes, minced (1 cup)
- Cooked legumes (1/2 cup)
- Spinach fronds (2 gallons)
- Red onion, thinly diced (1/4 cup)
- Feta cheese, shredded (2 tbsp)

- Olive oil (1 tbsp)
- Lemon juice (1 tbsp)

PREPARATION:
1. Toss roasted sweet potatoes, chickpeas, spinach, and red onion in a basin.
2. Sprinkle with crumbled feta.
3. Drizzle with olive oil and lemon juice.

NUTRITIONAL VALUE:
- Protein: 10g
- Healthy Fats: 8g
- Fiber: 6g

Cooking Time: 25 minutes

7. Salmon and Asparagus Foil Pack
INGREDIENTS:
- Salmon tenderloin (6 ounce)
- Asparagus segments (1 cup)
- Lemon segments (2)
- Olive oil (1 tbsp)
- Garlic, minced (1 tsp)
- Dill, minced (1 tsp)

PREPARATION:
1. Place salmon on a piece of foil.
2. Arrange asparagus around the salmon.

3. Drizzle with olive oil, scatter minced garlic, and distribute minced dill over the salmon and asparagus.

4. Place lemon segments on top.

5. Seal the foil into a bundle and bake in the oven until salmon is cooked.

NUTRITIONAL VALUE:

- Protein: 30g - Healthy Fats: 15g
- Fiber: 4g

Cooking Time: 20 minutes

8. Mushroom and Spinach Omelette

INGREDIENTS:

- Eggs (2)
- Mushrooms, diced (1/2 cup)
- Fresh spinach leaves (1 cup)
- Feta cheese, shredded (2 tbsp)
- Olive oil (1 tsp)
- Salt and pepper to flavor

PREPARATION:

1. Whisk eggs in a basin and season with salt and pepper.

2. In a skillet, sauté mushrooms and spinach in olive oil.

3. Pour whisked eggs over the vegetables.

4. Sprinkle crumbled feta on top.

5. Cook until the eggs are set and the underside is caramelized.

NUTRITIONAL VALUE:
- Protein: 18g - Healthy Fats: 12g

Cooking Time: 10 minutes

9. Tofu and Vegetable Brown Rice Bowl
INGREDIENTS:
- Firm tofu, diced (4 ounce)
- Brown rice, prepared (1 cup)
- Broccoli florets (1/2 cup)
- Carrots, julienned (1/4 cup)
- Snap peas (1/4 cup)
- Low-sodium soy sauce (2 tbsp)
- Sesame oil (1 tsp)
- Ginger, minced (1 tsp)

PREPARATION:
1. Press tofu to remove excess water and cube.
2. In a wok, stir-fry tofu until golden.
3. Add broccoli, carrots, and snap peas.
4. Pour in soy sauce, sesame oil, and grated ginger.
5. Serve over prepared brown rice.

NUTRITIONAL VALUE:
- Protein: 15g

- Healthy Fats: 7g
- Fiber: 6g

Cooking Time: 15 minutes

10. Black Bean and Avocado Wrap

INGREDIENTS:
- Whole grain tortilla (1)
- Black beans, strained and rinsed (1/2 cup)
- Avocado, diced (1/2)
- Cherry tomatoes, divided (1/4 cup)
- Red onion, minced (2 tbsp)
- Cilantro, minced (1 tbsp)
- Lime juice (1 tbsp)

PREPARATION:
1. Warm the whole grain tortilla.
2. Mash black beans and distribute on the tortilla.
3. Layer with avocado segments, cherry tomatoes, red onion, and cilantro.
4. Drizzle with lime juice.
5. Wrap and secure with toothpicks if required.

NUTRITIONAL VALUE:
- Protein: 10g
- Healthy Fats: 8g
- Fiber: 8g

Dinner Wonders: Satisfying and Nourishing Suppers

1. Grilled Salmon with Lemon and Dill

INGREDIENTS:
- 4 salmon fillets (6 ounces each)
- Fresh dill, chopped
- Lemon, sliced
- Olive oil
- Salt and pepper

PREPARATION:
1. Preheat the barbecue.
2. Rub salmon fillets with olive oil, garnish with minced dill, and season with salt and pepper.
3. Grill for 4-6 minutes per side or until the salmon is heated through.
4. Serve with fresh lemon segments.

NUTRITIONAL VALUE:
- Rich in omega-3 fatty acids.
- High in protein.

Cooking Time: 10-12 minutes

2. Turkey and Quinoa Stuffed Peppers

INGREDIENTS:
- 1 lb ground turkey
- 1 cup quinoa, boiled
- Bell peppers (4-6, halved)
- Onion, diced
- Garlic, minced
- Tomato sauce
- Italian seasoning
- Salt and pepper

PREPARATION:
1. Preheat the oven to 375°F (190°C).
2. Cook ground turkey with diced onion and minced garlic until browned.
3. Mix cooked quinoa, tomato sauce, Italian seasoning, salt, and pepper.
4. Stuff divided peppers with the turkey-quinoa mixture.
5. Bake for 25-30 minutes.

NUTRITIONAL VALUE:
- Lean protein from turkey.
- Quinoa provides fiber and essential nutrients.

Cooking Time: 30-35 minutes

3. Baked Cod with Herbed Cauliflower Mash

INGREDIENTS:
- Cod fillets (4, 6 ounces each)
- Cauliflower (1 head)
- Fresh parsley, chopped
- Garlic, minced
- Olive oil
- Lemon juice
- Salt and pepper

PREPARATION:
1. Preheat the oven to 400°F (200°C).
2. Place cod fillets on a baking sheet, drizzle with olive oil, minced garlic, and lemon juice. Season with salt and pepper.
3. Bake for 15-20 minutes.
4. Steam and puree cauliflower, combine with minced parsley, salt, and pepper.
5. Serve the cod over cauliflower puree.

Nutritional Value:
- Cod is an excellent source of lean protein.
- Cauliflower is low in calories and high in fiber.

Cooking Time: 20-25 minutes

4. Vegetarian Chickpea and Spinach Curry

INGREDIENTS:
- Chickpeas (2 cans, strained)
- Spinach (1 bundle)
- Onion, minced
- Tomatoes (2, diced)
- Coconut milk
- Curry seasonings
- Turmeric
- Ginger, minced
- Garlic, minced

PREPARATION:
1. In a pan, sauté diced onion, grated ginger, and minced garlic until translucent.
2. Add diced tomatoes, curry powder, and turmeric. Cook until tomatoes break down.
3. Add drained legumes and coconut milk. Simmer for 15 minutes.
4. Stir in fresh spinach until wilted.

NUTRITIONAL VALUE:
- Chickpeas provide protein and fiber.
- Spinach is abundant in iron and micronutrients.

Cooking Time: 25-30 minutes

5. Grilled Chicken Salad with Avocado

INGREDIENTS:
- Chicken breasts (2, boneless and skinless)
- Mixed salad vegetables
- Cherry tomatoes, halved
- Avocado, sliced - Olive oil
- Balsamic vinegar
- Dijon mustard
- Salt and pepper

PREPARATION:
1. Season chicken breasts with salt and pepper, grill until heated through.
2. In a basin, combine mixed greens, cherry tomatoes, and sliced avocado.
3. In a small basin, whisk together olive oil, balsamic vinegar, and Dijon mustard for vinaigrette.
4. Slice seared chicken and position on top of the salad.
5. Drizzle with the vinaigrette.

NUTRITIONAL VALUE:
- Lean protein from chicken.
- Avocado provides healthful nutrients.

Cooking Time: 15-20 minutes

6. Stir-Fried Tofu with Broccoli and Brown Rice

INGREDIENTS:
- Firm tofu (1 block, diced)
- Broccoli florets
- Brown rice (2 cups, boiled)
- Soy sauce
- Sesame oil
- Garlic, minced
- Ginger, minced
- Green scallions, minced

PREPARATION:
1. In a wok, stir-fry cubed tofu until golden.
2. Add minced garlic and grated ginger, stir-fry until aromatic.
3. Add broccoli florets and continue to stir-fry.
4. Drizzle with soy sauce and sesame oil.
5. Serve over prepared brown rice, garnish with minced green scallions.

NUTRITIONAL VALUE:
- Tofu provides plant-based protein.
- Broccoli is abundant in micronutrients and fiber.

Cooking Time: 20-25 minutes

7. Salmon and Asparagus Foil Packets

INGREDIENTS:
- Salmon fillets (4, 6 ounces each)
- Asparagus spears
- Lemon, sliced
- Garlic, minced
- Olive oil
- Dill, chopped - Salt and pepper

PREPARATION:
1. Preheat the oven to 375°F (190°C).
2. Place salmon fillets on individual foil sheets.
3. Arrange
1. Preheat the barbecue.
2. Rub salmon fillets with olive oil, garnish with minced dill, and season with salt and pepper.
3. Grill for 4-6 minutes per side or until the salmon is heated through.
4. Serve with fresh lemon segments.

NUTRITIONAL VALUE:
- Rich in omega-3 fatty acids.
- High in protein.

Cooking Time: 10-12 minutes

8. Mushroom and Lentil Stuffed Bell Peppers

INGREDIENTS:
- Bell peppers (4-6, halved)
- Lentils (1 cup, prepared)
- Mushrooms, minced
- Onion, minced
- Garlic, minced
- Tomato sauce
- Italian seasoning
- Salt and pepper

PREPARATION:
1. Preheat the oven to 375°F (190°C).
2. Sauté diced onion and minced garlic until translucent.
3. Add sliced mushrooms and simmer until tender.
4. Mix cooked legumes, tomato sauce, Italian seasoning, salt, and pepper.
5. Stuff divided peppers with the lentil-mushroom mixture.
6. Bake for 25-30 minutes.

NUTRITIONAL VALUE:
- Lentils provide plant-based protein and fiber.
- Bell peppers are abundant in minerals.

Cooking Time: 30-35 minutes

9. Shrimp and Quinoa Stir-Fry

INGREDIENTS:
- Shrimp (1 lb, skinned and deveined)
- Quinoa (2 cups, prepared)
- Broccoli florets
- Carrots, julienned
- Soy sauce
- Sesame oil
- Garlic, minced
- Ginger, minced
- Green scallions, minced

PREPARATION:
1. In a wok, stir-fry shrimp until scarlet and opaque.
2. Add minced garlic and grated ginger, stir-fry until aromatic.
3. Add broccoli florets and julienned carrots, continue to stir-fry.
4. Drizzle with soy sauce and sesame oil.
5. Mix in cooked quinoa and garnish with minced green scallions.

NUTRITIONAL VALUE:
- Shrimp is a low-calorie source of protein.
- Quinoa provides essential amino acids and fiber.

10. Baked Vegetable and Chicken Casserole

INGREDIENTS:
- Chicken thighs (4, bone-in and skin-on)
- Sweet potatoes, skinned and diced
- Brussels sprouts, halved
- Red onion, sliced
- Olive oil
- Rosemary, chopped
- Garlic, minced
- Salt and pepper

PREPARATION:
1. Preheat the oven to 375°F (190°C).
2. In a large bowl, combine diced sweet potatoes, divided Brussels sprouts, and sliced red onion with olive oil, chopped rosemary, minced garlic, salt, and pepper.
3. Place chicken thighs on top of the vegetable mélange.
4. Bake for 40-45 minutes or until chicken is warmed through.

NUTRITIONAL VALUE:
- Chicken thighs provide protein and healthful lipids.

- Sweet potatoes and Brussels sprouts offer micronutrients and fiber.

Cooking Time: 40-45 Minutes

Snack Attack: Healthy Bites Between Meals

1. Avocado and Tomato Salsa

Ingredients:
- 1 mature avocado, diced
- 1 cup cherry tomatoes, diced
- 1/4 cup red onion, finely minced
- Fresh cilantro, chopped
- Lime juice, to taste
- Salt and pepper, to flavor

Preparation:
- In a basin, combine minced avocado, tomatoes, red onion, and cilantro.
- Add lime juice, salt, and pepper.
- Mix gradually and serve.
- Nutritional Value: Rich in healthful lipids, fiber, and antioxidants.

Cooking Time: 10 minutes.

2. Greek Yogurt and Berry Parfait

INGREDIENTS:

- 1 cup Greek yogurt
- Mixed berries (blueberries, strawberries, raspberries)
- 2 teaspoons cereal
- Honey, to flavor

PREPARATION:

- Layer Greek yogurt, assorted berries, and granola in a glass.
- Drizzle with honey.
- Repeat layers.

NUTRITIONAL VALUE:

- High in protein, probiotics, and antioxidants.

Cooking Time: 5 minutes.

3. Roasted Chickpeas:

INGREDIENTS:

- 1 can (15 lb) legumes, drained and rinsed
- 1 tablespoon olive oil
- 1 teaspoon cumin - 1 teaspoon paprika
- Salt, to flavor

PREPARATION:

- Preheat oven to 400°F (200°C).

- Toss chickpeas with olive oil, cumin, paprika, and salt.
- Roast in the oven for 20-25 minutes until crusty.

NUTRITIONAL VALUE:
- Good source of protein and fiber.

Cooking Time: 25 minutes.

4. Cucumber and Hummus Bites
INGREDIENTS:
- Cucumber, cut
- Hummus
- Cherry tomatoes, divided
- Fresh dill, for garnish

PREPARATION:
- Spread hummus on cucumber segments.
- Top with cherry tomato halves.
- Garnish with fresh dill.

NUTRITIONAL VALUE:
- Low-calorie, hydrating, and rich in vitamins.

Cooking Time: 10 minutes.

5. Baked Apple Chips
INGREDIENTS:
- 2 pears, thinly cut
- Cinnamon, to flavor

PREPARATION:
- Preheat oven to 200°F (95°C).
- Arrange apple segments on a baking tray.
- Sprinkle with cinnamon.
- Bake for 2-3 hours until brown.

NUTRITIONAL VALUE:
- High in fiber and natural flavor.

Cooking Time: 2-3 hours.

6. Edamame with Sea Salt
INGREDIENTS:
- 1 cup edamame, steamed
- Sea salt, to flavor

PREPARATION:
- Steam edamame until tender.
- Sprinkle with sea salt.
- Toss to saturate.

NUTRITIONAL VALUE:
- Rich in protein, fiber, and essential nutrients.

Cooking Time: 5 minutes.

7. Kale Chips

INGREDIENTS:
- Fresh kale, divided into bite-sized segments
- Olive oil
- Garlic granules, to flavor
- Nutritional yeast, to flavor

PREPARATION:
- Preheat oven to 350°F (175°C).
- Toss kale with olive oil, garlic powder, and nutritional yeast.
- Bake until golden, about 10-15 minutes.

NUTRITIONAL VALUE:
- Low-calorie, rich in vitamins and minerals.

Cooking Time: 15 minutes.

8. Mango and Chili Lime Tajin

INGREDIENTS:
- Mango, cut
- Tajin seasoning
- Lime juice, to flavor

PREPARATION:
- Arrange mango segments on a platter.
- Sprinkle with Tajin seasoning.

- Drizzle with lime juice.

NUTRITIONAL VALUE:
- Vitamin C-rich, with a hint of spice.

Cooking Time: 5 minutes.

9. Caprese Skewers
INGREDIENTS:
- Cherry tomatoes
- Fresh mozzarella balls
- Basil fronds
- Balsamic glaze

PREPARATION:
- Thread cherry tomatoes, mozzarella spheres, and basil leaves onto skewers.
- Drizzle with balsamic marinade.

NUTRITIONAL VALUE:
- Provides healthful lipids and antioxidants.

Cooking Time: 10 minutes.

10. Almond Butter and Banana Rice Cakes
INGREDIENTS:
- Rice cakes
- Almond butter

- Banana, sliced
- Chia seeds, for garnish

PREPARATION:
- Spread almond butter on rice patties.
- Top with banana segments.
- Sprinkle with chia seeds.

NUTRITIONAL VALUE:
- Balanced with healthful lipids and natural flavor.

Cooking Time: 5 minutes.

Conclusion

In conclusion, we've gone on a path to improve liver health through a deliberate selection of recipes meant to nourish and support people navigating the challenges of fatty liver disorders. The variety of meals given here is more than just about maintaining the body; it's a celebration of flavors, textures, and nutritional richness tailored to the special demands of a liver-friendly diet.

We looked at a variety of foods, from nutrient-dense veggies and lean proteins to entire grains and healthy fats. Each dish has been designed not only to please the palate, but also to adhere to the principles of a diet that is beneficial to controlling or correcting fatty liver disorders. The attention to nutritional content, cooking methods, and portion sizes guarantees that these dishes provide a harmonic balance that promotes general well-being.

As you go through this cookbook, keep in mind that eating fatty liver-friendly foods is more than just a culinary decision; it's a commitment to your health. The recipes on this page are intended to promote a long-term lifestyle change, encouraging you to recognize the influence of nutrition on your body. By eating these tasty and nutritious meals, you'll be on your way to enhanced liver function, more energy, and overall vitality.

Motivation is essential in every transforming journey. So, to you, the reader, I provide this particular incentive: Your health is an investment that will last a lifetime, and every nutritional choice you make is a step toward a healthier, more vibrant you. Accept the pleasure of fueling your body with nutritious, liver-friendly meals. Celebrate the tastes and the trip, knowing that each bite helps you feel better. Remember that modest adjustments have big outcomes, and your dedication to this lifestyle change is a tremendous act of self-care. May this cookbook serve as your guide, allowing you to experience not just the delectable recipes contained inside its pages, but also the transforming path toward a healthier, happier self. Cheers to a healthy life and a well-nourished liver!

Contact Us

Dear valued reader,

First and foremost, I would like to express my sincere gratitude for choosing my book FATTY LIVER DIET COOKBOOK FOR BEGINNERS as your guide. I hope that you found the content helpful, informative, and enjoyable to read.

THE BONUS - SPECIAL RECIPE TRACKER is in the next page.

I also want to remind you that your feedback is important to me. I would love to hear your thoughts, observations, questions and suggestions about the book, so that I can continue to improve and provide you with even more valuable content in the future.

You can contact me through this email: Coreyhelpdesk@gmail.com

Thank you once again for choosing my book, and I look forward to hearing from you soon!

Best regards,
Corey Pearce

THIS PAGE WAS INTENTIONALLY LEFT BLANK

THE BONUS - SPECIAL
RECIPE TRACKER

SPECIAL MEAL TRACKER

DATE:...............................

			SNACKS
MONDAY	BREAKFAST		
	LUNCH		
	DINNER		
TUESDAY	BREAKFAST		
	LUNCH		
	DINNER		
WEDNESDAY	BREAKFAST		
	LUNCH		
	DINNER		
THURSDAY	BREAKFAST		
	LUNCH		
	DINNER		
FRIDAY	BREAKFAST		NOTE
	LUNCH		
	DINNER		
SATURDAY	BREAKFAST		
	LUNCH		
	DINNER		
SUNDAY	BREAKFAST		
	LUNCH		
	DINNER		

SPECIAL MEAL TRACKER

DATE:................................

MONDAY	BREAKFAST	
	LUNCH	
	DINNER	
TUESDAY	BREAKFAST	
	LUNCH	
	DINNER	
WEDNESDAY	BREAKFAST	
	LUNCH	
	DINNER	
THURSDAY	BREAKFAST	
	LUNCH	
	DINNER	
FRIDAY	BREAKFAST	
	LUNCH	
	DINNER	
SATURDAY	BREAKFAST	
	LUNCH	
	DINNER	
SUNDAY	BREAKFAST	
	LUNCH	
	DINNER	

SNACKS

NOTE

SPECIAL MEAL TRACKER

DATE:................................

			SNACKS
MONDAY	BREAKFAST		
	LUNCH		
	DINNER		
TUESDAY	BREAKFAST		
	LUNCH		
	DINNER		
WEDNESDAY	BREAKFAST		
	LUNCH		
	DINNER		
THURSDAY	BREAKFAST		
	LUNCH		
	DINNER		
FRIDAY	BREAKFAST		
	LUNCH		NOTE
	DINNER		
SATURDAY	BREAKFAST		
	LUNCH		
	DINNER		
SUNDAY	BREAKFAST		
	LUNCH		
	DINNER		

SPECIAL MEAL TRACKER

DATE:...............................

MONDAY	BREAKFAST	
	LUNCH	
	DINNER	
TUESDAY	BREAKFAST	
	LUNCH	
	DINNER	
WEDNESDAY	BREAKFAST	
	LUNCH	
	DINNER	
THURSDAY	BREAKFAST	
	LUNCH	
	DINNER	
FRIDAY	BREAKFAST	
	LUNCH	
	DINNER	
SATURDAY	BREAKFAST	
	LUNCH	
	DINNER	
SUNDAY	BREAKFAST	
	LUNCH	
	DINNER	

SNACKS

NOTE

SPECIAL MEAL TRACKER

DATE:................................

MONDAY	BREAKFAST	
	LUNCH	
	DINNER	
TUESDAY	BREAKFAST	
	LUNCH	
	DINNER	
WEDNESDAY	BREAKFAST	
	LUNCH	
	DINNER	
THURSDAY	BREAKFAST	
	LUNCH	
	DINNER	
FRIDAY	BREAKFAST	
	LUNCH	
	DINNER	
SATURDAY	BREAKFAST	
	LUNCH	
	DINNER	
SUNDAY	BREAKFAST	
	LUNCH	
	DINNER	

SNACKS

NOTE

SPECIAL MEAL TRACKER

DATE:................................

MONDAY	BREAKFAST	
	LUNCH	
	DINNER	
TUESDAY	BREAKFAST	
	LUNCH	
	DINNER	
WEDNESDAY	BREAKFAST	
	LUNCH	
	DINNER	
THURSDAY	BREAKFAST	
	LUNCH	
	DINNER	
FRIDAY	BREAKFAST	
	LUNCH	
	DINNER	
SATURDAY	BREAKFAST	
	LUNCH	
	DINNER	
SUNDAY	BREAKFAST	
	LUNCH	
	DINNER	

SNACKS

NOTE

SPECIAL MEAL TRACKER

DATE:................................

			SNACKS
MONDAY	BREAKFAST		
	LUNCH		
	DINNER		
TUESDAY	BREAKFAST		
	LUNCH		
	DINNER		
WEDNESDAY	BREAKFAST		
	LUNCH		
	DINNER		
THURSDAY	BREAKFAST		
	LUNCH		
	DINNER		
FRIDAY	BREAKFAST		NOTE
	LUNCH		
	DINNER		
SATURDAY	BREAKFAST		
	LUNCH		
	DINNER		
SUNDAY	BREAKFAST		
	LUNCH		
	DINNER		

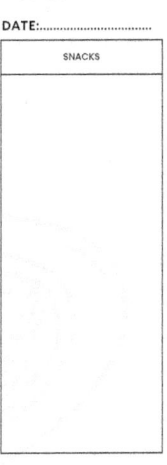
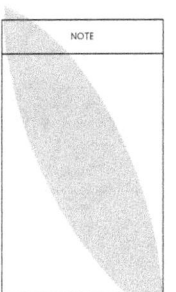

SPECIAL MEAL TRACKER

DATE:................................

MONDAY	BREAKFAST	
	LUNCH	
	DINNER	
TUESDAY	BREAKFAST	
	LUNCH	
	DINNER	
WEDNESDAY	BREAKFAST	
	LUNCH	
	DINNER	
THURSDAY	BREAKFAST	
	LUNCH	
	DINNER	
FRIDAY	BREAKFAST	
	LUNCH	
	DINNER	
SATURDAY	BREAKFAST	
	LUNCH	
	DINNER	
SUNDAY	BREAKFAST	
	LUNCH	
	DINNER	

SNACKS

NOTE

SPECIAL MEAL TRACKER

DATE:................................

			SNACKS
MONDAY	BREAKFAST		
	LUNCH		
	DINNER		
TUESDAY	BREAKFAST		
	LUNCH		
	DINNER		
WEDNESDAY	BREAKFAST		
	LUNCH		
	DINNER		
THURSDAY	BREAKFAST		
	LUNCH		
	DINNER		
FRIDAY	BREAKFAST		NOTE
	LUNCH		
	DINNER		
SATURDAY	BREAKFAST		
	LUNCH		
	DINNER		
SUNDAY	BREAKFAST		
	LUNCH		
	DINNER		

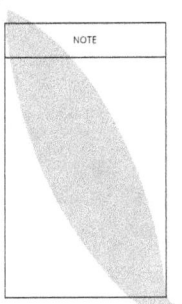

SPECIAL MEAL TRACKER

DATE:................................

MONDAY	BREAKFAST	
	LUNCH	
	DINNER	
TUESDAY	BREAKFAST	
	LUNCH	
	DINNER	
WEDNESDAY	BREAKFAST	
	LUNCH	
	DINNER	
THURSDAY	BREAKFAST	
	LUNCH	
	DINNER	
FRIDAY	BREAKFAST	
	LUNCH	
	DINNER	
SATURDAY	BREAKFAST	
	LUNCH	
	DINNER	
SUNDAY	BREAKFAST	
	LUNCH	
	DINNER	

SNACKS

NOTE